I0702904

THE 80/20 DIET FOR EASY WEIGHT LOSS

A No-Stress Meal Plan to Burn Fat at Your Own Pace Without Feeling Guilty About Indulging in Your Favorite Foods

Joe Miller, RD

Copyright Page

Copyright © 2024 Joe Miller, RD

All rights reserved. No part of this publication may be reproduced, distributed, or transmitted in any form or by any means, including photocopying, recording, or other electronic or mechanical methods, without the prior written permission of the publisher, except in the case of brief quotation embodied in critical reviews and certain other non-commercial uses permitted by copyright law.

Table of Contents

INTRODUCTION

The Pareto Principle, an economic guideline, posits that 80% of outcomes or outputs arise from 20% of inputs or causes. This principle forms the foundation of the 80/20 diet, which suggests dedicating 80% of dietary efforts to healthy eating and allowing the remaining 20% for indulgence or rest. Rather than dictating strict rules for food consumption, the 80/20 diet serves as more of a philosophy, leaving the implementation up to individual preferences.

Maintaining a consistently healthy diet can be challenging, particularly when compared to other, more rigid diet regimens. The 80/20 rule stands out as a simpler and more adaptable approach. If you're curious about exploring the 80/20 rule diet, it offers an adjustable eating plan that doesn't necessitate complete abstinence from indulgent foods, like cheese.

Diets often involve significant sacrifices, making it difficult for those attempting to lose weight. The very term "diet" can trigger hunger pangs, leading to overindulgence in high-calorie, fatty meals. In contrast, the 80/20 rule provides a refreshingly easy approach. It suggests prioritizing healthful, nourishing meals 80% of the time, allowing for the enjoyment of less healthy options during the remaining 20%. This more relaxed eating style rejects the notion of rigid dieting, promoting a balanced diet that accommodates occasional treats in moderation.

While altering dietary habits can be challenging, potentially resulting in weight loss, increased energy, and reduced disease risk, adhering to healthy choices throughout the day may seem overwhelming. The 80/20 rule dismisses this notion, asserting that strict adherence to a healthy diet at every meal is unnecessary.

Key to the 80/20 approach is patience, emphasizing the significance of consistent actions. Recognizing that occasional indulgence is a natural part of real-world scenarios, this approach offers a more realistic perspective on healthy eating. The 80/20 plan presents a viable alternative to completely eliminating junk food or sweets, providing an opportunity to enjoy favorite foods in moderation. Discover whether this approach aligns with your goals and learn about its workings by delving into the details.

You might already be familiar with the 80/20 Diet, which, instead of imposing strict dietary rules, operates more like a flexible philosophy towards food. Rooted in the Pareto Principle from economics, stating that a small portion is responsible for a large outcome, this diet encourages aiming for healthy eating 80% of the time while allowing a bit more flexibility for the remaining 20%.

Adhering to a healthy diet can be challenging, right? That's where the 80/20 rule steps in, showcasing its simplicity and adaptability in contrast to more rigid approaches. So, what's the essence of the 80/20 Diet? The good news is, you don't have to entirely eliminate your favorite meals. For instance, you can still savor cheese, as long as it falls within the 20% flexibility zone – no need to cut it out entirely.

Embarking on weight loss often involves difficult dietary sacrifices. The mere mention of the term "diet" might trigger cravings for something sweet and unhealthy. Enter the 80/20 rule, a refreshing departure from conventional dieting norms. The basic idea is to prioritize nutritious, healthful foods for 80% of your meals, reserving the remaining 20% for less nutritious options. Bid farewell to the strict regulations of traditional diets and welcome moderation and balance.

Initiating changes in eating habits for weight loss, enhanced energy, and improved health can be intimidating. Some diets demand flawless adherence all the time, but the 80/20 Diet rejects this "all or nothing" approach. It acknowledges that occasional indulgence is acceptable, recognizing the realities of life.

With the 80/20 method, patience is the cornerstone. The premise is that consistent, reasonable actions have a more significant impact than striving for perfection. So, it's perfectly fine to treat yourself every now and then. This approach considers the practicalities of everyday life, offering a realistic perspective on healthy eating.

If you've grown weary of rigid and punishing diet plans, the 80/20 approach might be a breath of fresh air. You can still enjoy your favorite foods without entirely eliminating them. Curious about its workings? Dive into the details for a more sensible and well-rounded strategy to achieve your dietary and health goals.

The Basics of the 80/20 Principle

Discover a fresh perspective on maintaining a harmonious work-life balance through an in-depth exploration of the 80/20 Principle, which we'll now delve into. At its core, this principle posits that a small percentage of inputs (20%) yield a substantial portion of outputs (80%). According

to the 80/20 rule, prioritize healthy eating for 80%
of the time while allowing a flexible 20%.

The hallmark of the 80/20 Principle is its
adaptability. Instead of being a rigid set of rules
governing every action, it serves as a flexible
philosophy that accommodates personal
preferences. The key advice is to focus on healthy
eating most of the time but also permit occasional
indulgences.

Achieving a consistently healthy diet can be
challenging, and the 80/20 rule recognizes this
reality. Unlike other diet plans, it offers both
flexibility and simplicity. Acknowledging the
natural inclination to find comfort in familiar

foods or break away from routine, it provides a practical and achievable framework.

Contrary to misconceptions, the 80/20 rule is not about deprivation. It introduces an enjoyable transition to a healthier lifestyle by allowing the consumption of preferred foods. Maintaining consistent behavior over time necessitates a blend of self-control and adaptability, and this method strikes a favorable balance between the two.

In essence, the 80/20 rule marks a refreshing departure from traditional dieting approaches. It advocates for a balanced, healthy lifestyle rather than one with stringent rules. Embracing this philosophy means committing to a long-term approach that accommodates the fluctuations of life. Striving for balance on your journey to health holds more significance than aiming for perfection.

Benefits and Science Behind the Approach

The 80/20 diet plan offers a balanced approach to dieting, allowing you to enjoy some of your favorite, less healthy foods in moderation. Let's face it, dieting can be tough. Anyone who has tried to lose weight knows how hard it is to give up beloved foods and stick to a strict regimen.

Even the word "diet" can make us feel deprived, often leading to overindulgence in high-calorie, high-fat foods.

Here's some good news: the 80/20 Diet is a new eating plan that lets you indulge in your favorite treats as long as you eat healthily most of the time. One great aspect of this diet is that it alleviates the guilt we often feel when enjoying non-diet foods like cupcakes, cookies, and ice cream.

Allowing yourself to occasionally enjoy a favorite food can help prevent binge eating. Overly restrictive eating rarely makes anyone happy because it's extremely challenging. Some level of control is beneficial, but setting too many rules can lead to failure and starting over from scratch.

The 80/20 Diet addresses both the physical and mental aspects of weight loss and could be a practical, sustainable way to lose weight and stay healthy. It's always a good idea to consult a registered dietitian or healthcare professional before making significant changes to your diet.

This way of eating has many benefits:

Easy to follow: The 80/20 diet isn't a restrictive, all-or-nothing plan. You include all your meals and treats, just adjusting their proportions.

No counting: There's no need for food tracking apps or diaries to count calories or carbs.

No forbidden foods: On the 80/20 diet, no food is off-limits. You can enjoy everything you like, just not all the time.

No deprivation: If you're at a party or a special event, you can still enjoy indulgences like restaurant meals or birthday cake.

Promotes healthy habits: Eating nutritious foods 80% of the time helps you adopt healthy cooking methods and smart grocery shopping strategies.

Flexible for any dietary needs: This diet can accommodate various dietary restrictions, whether you're gluten-free, vegan, diabetic, or have allergies.

CHAPTER 2
Is the 80/20 Diet Right for You?

The 80/20 diet is flexible and not too strict, making it a good fit with expert advice on healthy eating. It's similar to other slow-and-steady weight loss plans. For example, the MyPlate guidelines from the U.S. Department of Agriculture (USDA) recommend balanced meals with reasonable portions of grains, lean meats, fruits, vegetables, and low-fat dairy, which matches the 80/20 diet's ideas.

The USDA suggests women should aim for about 1500 calories a day and men around 2000 calories a day to lose weight. These amounts can change based on your age, sex, activity level, and weight.

The 80/20 diet doesn't give a specific calorie count, which is one reason it's so easy to stick to.

With the 80/20 diet, you focus on eating healthy foods 80% of the time and allow yourself to enjoy your favorite treats the other 20% of the time. This balance helps you avoid feeling deprived while still making progress towards your weight loss goals.

How the 80/20 Diet Affects Cholesterol, Weight, Mood, and Energy

To enhance cholesterol levels, energy, weight management, mood, and overall health, the 80/20 diet serves as an excellent starting point. This section delves into the distinctive approach of this method in addressing these vital aspects.

The 80/20 diet places a spotlight on nutrient-dense foods that promote heart health, thereby positively influencing cholesterol levels. Opting for a diet rich in whole grains, vegetables, fruits, and lean proteins contributes to the maintenance of a healthy lipid profile and the reduction of cholesterol levels. Elevating cardiovascular health is achievable by incorporating heart-healthy choices into the majority of nutrient-rich meals, constituting 80% of the dietary plan.

A standout feature of the 80/20 diet lies in its unique approach to weight management. It advocates for a sustainable and pragmatic eating style by advocating a balance between nutritious food choices and occasional indulgences. This flexibility proves instrumental for those seeking to maintain a healthy weight, as it fosters adherence to the plan without the common feeling of deprivation associated with more restrictive diets. Following the 80/20 principle allows for enjoyment without compromising health.

Recognizing the profound impact of nutrition on mental and emotional well-being, the 80/20 diet incorporates a strategy that considers the psychological aspect of eating. Permitting occasional indulgences fosters a healthy relationship with food, alleviating feelings of constraint. With a focus on nutrient-rich foods constituting the majority of the diet, the plan contributes to steady blood sugar levels, promoting mental stability and overall well-being.

Energy levels, both mental and physical, experience a direct positive impact from the 80/20 diet. The predominance of nutritious, whole foods in the meals provides sustained energy throughout the day. Supplementing the diet with a diverse array of vitamins, minerals, and macronutrients enhances energy levels and resilience to fatigue. The 20% allowance for indulgences recognizes the importance of enjoying food for pleasure, contributing to a holistic and long-term boost in energy levels.

Essentially, the 80/20 diet views overall health and wellness holistically, beyond a set of rigid food rules. By intentionally balancing nutrient-rich choices with occasional pleasures, individuals can cultivate a nutritional habit that is both sustainable and enjoyable, positively impacting cholesterol, weight, mood, and energy levels.

Jacques Pépin's Criques (Crispy Potato Pancakes)

Ingredients You Need

For the pancakes:

2 cups (400g) peeled and cubed (about 1-inch) Russet potatoes

1 cup (100g) cubed (about 1-inch) white or yellow onion

2 cloves garlic, peeled

2 large eggs

2 tablespoons potato starch or all-purpose flour

1/2 teaspoon baking powder

1/2 teaspoon fine salt

1/2 teaspoon freshly ground black pepper

1/4 cup minced scallions

Peanut or canola oil, to sauté the pancakes

For the salad:

4 cups salad greens, like arugula or a mix

1 tablespoons extra-virgin olive oil

1 tablespoon red wine vinegar

Dash salt and freshly ground pepper

How to Make

Put the potatoes, onion, garlic, eggs, potato starch, baking powder, salt, and pepper in a food processor. Process for about 30 seconds to combine the ingredients well. The texture will be grainy. Stir or briefly pulse in the scallions.

Heat about 3 tablespoons oil in a large, nonstick skillet over high heat. When it is hot, add about 1/4 cup batter, spreading it out to form a pancake about 4 inches in diameter. Repeat this to have 4 pancakes cooking side by side in the pan. (If using a smaller pan, make multiple batches.) Cook the pancakes for about 3 minutes on each side over medium to high heat, fiddling with the heat as needed to make sure they don't burn before they cook through. They should be well browned and not squishy in the middle — you want to be sure the onions in the batter have a chance to cook through and lose their raw taste.

Transfer the pancakes to a wire rack so they don't get mushy on the underside. Continue making pancakes until all the batter is used, adding more oil to the pan as needed. Serve. (The criques are best fresh from the pan but can be made 1 to 2 hours ahead and reheated on a baking sheet in a 425° F oven for about 5 minutes before serving.)

To make the salad, toss the greens in a bowl with the olive oil, vinegar, and salt and pepper to taste. Divide among four plates and arrange the criques on top.

Leek and Greens Tart with Cornmeal Crust

Ingredients You Need

Cornmeal pastry dough

1 1/2 cups all purpose flour

1/2 cup cornmeal

1/2 teaspoon salt

1 tablespoon light brown sugar

1/2 teaspoon freshly ground nutmeg

12 tablespoons cold unsalted butter, cut into small pieces (yes, I know that's a lot, but just trust me, you'll be glad!)

1/4 cup ice cold water, plus a couple Tbs. more as necessary

Leeks and greens tart

1 bunch of kale, washed and tough stalks removed (you could also use another winter green, if you'd like, kale is just my favorite)

5 cloves of garlic, peeled but left whole

3 medium leeks, washed well and thinly sliced - just the white and light green portions

2 tablespoons olive oil

1 cup oacked grated Cantal cheese (or Gruyere)

juice of 1 lemon

1/2 cup mascarpone cheese

2 eggs

sea salt and fresh ground pepper

prepared cornmeal tart crust

How to Make

Cornmeal pastry dough

In a mixing bowl combine the flour, cornmeal, salt, sugar and nutmeg.

Add in the butter, then working quickly rub it in with your fingers or cut it in with a pastry cutter until it is mixed in and you have lumps about the size of peas. Stick this flour and butter mixture in the fridge for 10 minutes (this is a step that I discovered accidentally by being called away from the kitchen, and have found that it really enhances the final texture of the pastry).

Take the flour-butter mixture out of the fridge. Stir in the quarter cup water with a fork until the dough just comes together into a bunch of large dough clumps. Add more water 1 Tbs. at a time as needed to form the dough. Gather the pieces together and press them into a ball. Divide the dough into 2 pieces, one slightly lager than the other, flatten them into discs, wrap them in plastic wrap and refrigerate them at least 1 hour, and up to overnight.

When you are ready to make your tart, take the larger dough disc out of the fridge. If it is too hard to roll, let it sit at room temperature 5-10 minutes, but you don't want it to get too soft. On a lightly floured surface, roll the larger piece of dough out into a circle about 1/8 inch thick. Lightly drape the rolled dough over a 9-inch round tart pan, press it into the pan and trim the edges. Wait to roll out the other piece of dough until the tart is filled.

Line the bottom crust with parchment or foil and weight it. Bake in a 425F oven for 20 minutes. Remove from oven, remove the weights and lining, return to the oven and bake for another 5 minutes. Then, set aside.

Leeks and greens tart

Put kale and garlic cloves in a steamer basket and steam for 10 minutes. Allow to cool just enough to handle, then chop the kale well and smash the garlic to a paste.

In the meantime, heat the olive oil over medium heat in a large frying pan. When the oil is shimmering, add the leeks. Stir and cook for 5 minutes over medium, then turn the heat to medium low and cook until the leeks are a lovely soft golden pile, about another 20 minutes. Turn the heat back to medium, stir in the kale and garlic and cook for another 5 minutes until the flavors have mingled and any extra liquid has cooked off.

Transfer to a bowl. Allow to cool slightly, then stir in the Cantal cheese and lemon juice. At this point you can also preheat your oven to 350F. Taste the kale mixture and add salt and pepper to taste. Then stir in the eggs and mascarpone until everything is well combined.

Spread the vegetable and cheese mixture into the prepared tart crust. On a lightly floured surface, roll out the second piece of dough into a 9 inch circle (use a pie plate to trace and trim it into a perfect circle), cut a shape or slits in the top and lay this over the tart filling. You don't need to seal the top crust with the bottom, leaving a space gives the tart another air vent, and adds aesthetic interest. If you prefer, you could also use the second piece of dough to make a lattice-work top. Or, if you want an open topped tart, then just save the second piece of dough for something else (actually you can cut it into little squares and bake it and it makes awesome crackers!).

Place a rimmed baking sheet on the bottom shelf of your oven to catch any drips, and place the tart on the middle shelf. Bake for 50-60 minutes, or until the crust is golden brown and the filling is bubbly and fragrant. Allow to cool for at least 10 minutes before attempting to remove the tart pan rim.

Serve the tart warm or at room temperature.

Overnight Apple-Cinnamon French Toast

Ingredients You Need

1 pound loaf inexpensive supermarket French or Italian bread

8 large or extra large eggs, slightly beaten

3 1/2 cups skim milk

1/2 cup plus 3 tablespoons sugar, divided

1 1/2 teaspoons pure vanilla extract

5 to 6 apples, sliced thin (I like Golden Delicious)

1 1/2 teaspoons cinnamon

1 tablespoon butter (salted is fine), chopped

How to Make

Grease a 9-by 13-inch pan with butter or nonstick spray.

Cut the bread into 1 1/2-inch slices and pack them tightly into the prepared pan in one layer.

In a large bowl, stir together eggs, milk, 1/2 cup sugar, and vanilla. Pour half of this egg mixture over the bread slices.

Distribute the apple slices over the bread, and top with the remaining egg mixture.

In a small bowl, combine the remaining 3 tablespoons sugar and the cinnamon and sprinkle this mixture evenly over everything in the pan. Dot with butter.

Cover the whole thing and refrigerate overnight or for at least 6 hours.

The next day, or when ready to bake, preheat the oven to 350° F. Uncover the pan and bake for 50 to 60 minutes. Let stand for about 10 minutes, then cut into squares and serve warm (with maple syrup if you'd like) and enjoy!

Croissant French Toast

Ingredients You Need

2 large croissants

2 large eggs

Finely grated zest and juice of one orange

1/2 teaspoon vanilla extract

1 cup whole milk

1 cup good maple syrup

1 tablespoon Cointreau or Grand Marnier

2 tablespoons unsalted butter

Mascarpone for serving (optional)

How to Make

Using a serrated knife, carefully slice each croissant in half and set aside.

Whisk together the eggs, orange zest and juice, vanilla and milk in a large shallow pan or bowl. Meanwhile, warm the maple syrup in a small saucepan and stir in the Cointreau.

Set a large heavy skillet over medium heat and add 1 tablespoon of the butter. When it starts to foam, dip two of the croissant halves briefly in the egg and milk mixture, turning to coat both sides. (Do not leave them in the liquid, as they will become soggy.) Add them to the pan and cook, flipping once, until golden brown on both sides. Transfer to a plate and keep covered in a warm oven while you repeat with the rest of the croissants. Serve the french toast with the syrup, topping with a dollop of mascarpone if you like.

Frittata Affogata with Capers, Olives, and Anchovies

Ingredients You Need

For the sauce:

2 tablespoons extra-virgin olive oil

1/2 yellow onion, finely chopped

1/2 carrot, finely chopped

1/2 stalk of celery, finely chopped

400 grams tomatoes, fresh or canned, chopped (drain if canned)

2 tablespoons Italian parsley, chopped

2 tablespoons capers, coarsely chopped

4 anchovy fillets, coarsely chopped

7 Kalamata olives, coarsely chopped

salt and freshly ground black pepper to taste

1 pinch cayenne, or to taste

For the frittata:

4 eggs

1 tablespoon flour

salt and freshly ground pepper to taste

How to Make

In the small sauce pan heat 1 tablespoon of the olive oil. Add the onion, carrot, and celery and cook slowly until they just begin to brown. This will take about 15 minutes. Now add the tomatoes and parsley. Stir well and cook for 10 minutes. Add the capers, anchovies, and olives and stir well. Add salt and pepper to taste. Simmer the sauce for 5 minutes more, being careful not to let it scorch on the bottom. It should be thick. Set aside, covered, to keep it warm. (Note: You can make the sauce a day ahead and reheat it before serving.)

Beat the eggs in a bowl with salt and pepper. Beat in the flour until perfectly mixed. Heat the remaining 1 tablespoon of olive oil in a small frying pan. Pour in the beaten egg mixture. And allow to brown on one side. I find as the edges cook I can slide a spatula under so some of the uncooked egg flows beneath.

When the top is no longer runny, flip the frittata over and brown the other side. Cut the frittata into four or six pieces and place on individual plates. Pour the sauce over them. Reheat the sauce if needed.

"Moroccan Guacamole" Toasts with Fried Egg

Ingredients You Need

1 ripe avocado, halved and pitted

1/8 to 1/4 preserved lemon (including pulp) plus a little curing liquid, if desired

2 thick slices whole-grain bread

1 to 2 tablespoons olive oil

2 eggs

Pinch salt

Aleppo pepper or good-quality harissa as an accompaniment, if desired

lemon wedges, optional

How to Make

Make "guacamole:" Squeeze or scoop avocado flesh into a bowl. Mash lightly. Finely mince the cured lemon and add it to the avocado. Taste for seasoning; add a drizzle of the lemon curing liquid, plus a sprinkle of salt.

Toast your bread the way you like it. While the bread is toasting, warm the olive oil over a low flame in a non-stick pan. When it sizzles, break in two eggs and fry them to your desired donenesss

Spread avocado mixture on the bread, then top with eggs. Sprinkle yolks with Aleppo pepper or drizzle with harissa. Garnish with a wedge of lemon.

Breakfast is served!

Brussels Sprouts Hash & Eggs

Ingredients You Need

4 cups Brussels sprouts

Salt and pepper

1 tablespoon butter

3 cloves garlic

6 olives, finely chopped (any kind; we used kalamata olives)

2 eggs

Lemon juice

How to Make

Chop off the ends of the sprouts. Slice them in half, then finely shred each half. Place the shreds in a bowl and sprinkle with salt and pepper.

Melt the butter in a nonstick pan on medium-high heat. Swirl it around to coat the pan. Add the shredded Brussels sprouts and garlic, then leave it to cook for about 1 minute. Mix it up and toss it around. Add the olives and mix again.

Crack the eggs into opposite sides of the pan. Sprinkle them with salt and pepper. Pour in 2 tablespoons of water and cover with a lid. Let the eggs steam, undisturbed, for 2 minutes.

Once the whites of the eggs are cooked through, turn off the heat and sprinkle everything with lemon juice, to taste.

Spiced Millet Pilaf with Beetroot, Feta and Mint

Ingredients You Need

For the millet pilaf:

1 bunch baby beetroot (baby beets), leaves reserved

1/4 cup ghee or olive oil

2 teaspoons black mustard seeds

2 teaspoons yellow mustard seeds

2 teaspoons cumin seeds

1 large onion, finely chopped

2 garlic cloves, finely chopped

1 1/2 serrano chilies, finely chopped

3 to 4 curry leaves

1 teaspoon ground turmeric

1 1/2 cups hulled millet

1/2 cup cashew nuts, lightly toasted and roughly chopped

Cilantro and mint leaves, feta, and lemon wedges, to serve

For the mint and beetroot green pesto:

Trimmed leaves from the baby beetroot, washed

1 cup packed mint leaves

1/2 cup cashew nuts, toasted

1/2 serrano chili

1/3 cup extra-virgin olive oil

1/4 cup lemon juice

How to Make

For the millet pilaf:

Place beetroot into a saucepan, cover with water, and bring to the boil over high heat. Reduce heat to low and simmer for 20 to 25 minutes until tender. Remove from the heat, drain, and set aside until cool enough to handle. Peel the beetroot and cut into pieces.

Place ghee in a large saucepan over medium heat. Add the mustard seeds and cumin seeds. When the seeds start to pop, add the onion and cook, stirring, for 1 to 2 minutes, until tender. Add the garlic, chili, curry leaves, and turmeric, then cook, stirring, for another 30 seconds, or until fragrant. Stir in the millet, 1/2 teaspoon fine sea salt and cook, stirring, for 1 to 2 minutes to toast the grains. Pour in 3 cups cold water (it will splatter, so take care). Stir to combine and cover with a lid. Bring to the boil then reduce heat to low and simmer, covered, without stirring, for 20 minutes. Remove from the heat, leave the lid on and set aside for 5 minutes before fluffing up with a fork. Cover and keep warm until ready to serve.

To serve, stir in the cashews, cilantro, and mint. Spoon onto plates, top with chopped beetroot, crumble over feta, and drizzle with a little pesto (see recipe below). Serve with extra lemon wedges for squeezing over.

For the mint and beetroot green pesto:

Place all the ingredients in a small food processor and whiz to form a smooth paste. Season well. To make the pesto thinner, simply add a little more lemon juice and extra-virgin olive oil until it's the desired consistency. Set aside until ready to use.

Andrew Feinberg's Slow-Baked Broccoli Frittata

Ingredients You Need

10 large eggs

2 1/2 tablespoons grated Parmigiano Reggiano, plus more for serving

1 teaspoon kosher salt, plus more

40 turns of a black pepper mill

7 tablespoons extra-virgin olive oil, divided, plus more for serving

1 medium (1-pound) head of broccoli (4 cups once trimmed)

1/2 red onion, thinly sliced

1 heaping tablespoon chopped garlic

1/8 teaspoon plus 1 large pinch of dried red pepper flakes

1 squeeze fresh lemon juice, to taste

How to Make

Heat the oven to 400°F. In a large bowl, whisk the eggs, cheese, 1 teaspoon of the salt, and the black pepper; set aside.

Trim ½ inch off the stem of the broccoli. Using a knife, separate all the florets from the base, leaving the stem attached. Cut the florets in half (you can cut any especially large ones into quarters so all are evenly sized).

In a 10- to 11-inch oven-safe sauté pan over medium-high heat, warm ¼ cup of the oil. Cook the broccoli, mostly undisturbed to develop a nice brown color on one side, then turn and season with salt. Transfer the pan to the oven and roast for 10 to 15 minutes, until tender.

In another 10- to 11-inch sauté pan over medium-high heat, warm 2 tablespoons of the oil. Add the onions, season with salt, and cook, stirring occasionally, for 3 to 5 minutes, until lightly browned.

Once the broccoli is roasted, return the pan to the stovetop and reduce the oven temperature to 300°F.

Heat the broccoli over medium heat, then add the garlic, red pepper flakes, and 1 tablespoon of the oil. Carefully cook, stirring occasionally, for 1 minute, so as not to burn the garlic. Add the onions to the broccoli and mix well to combine. Add the egg mixture, increase the heat to high, and cook for 30 seconds.

Transfer the pan to the oven and bake for 25 to 30 minutes, until the eggs are just set. Using a rubber spatula, turn out the frittata onto a serving plate. Squeeze the lemon juice over the top, drizzle with oil, and sprinkle with Parmigiano Reggiano.

Josh Ozersky's 3-Minute Hash Browns

Ingredients You Need

Potatoes (about 1/2 medium potato per person)

Salted butter

Kosher salt

How to Make

Take a big pan, sizzle some salted butter in it, and just when the foaming subsides, coarsely grate an unpeeled potato over it on the large holes of a box grater. The potato, unmolested will still have all its starchy essence and the flavor that conveys. Do it sparingly, so that you see as much pan as potato; don't pile it up anywhere. Ozersky used a 12-inch skillet and rarely did more than half a medium potato at a time. (Alternately, you can grate the potato on the side if you need to brace the grater against the counter, then sprinkle in your latticework by hand.)

Once the potato hits the pan, salt it. The reason you want there to be so much space is to give the steam somewhere to go. Potatoes need to shrink and shrivel, concentrating their taste down and replacing their water with precious fat. They can't do that if they're being jammed in next to each other like the crowd at a Motorhead concert. Give them room and let them bind with each other as the starch comes out. Amazingly, the shreds will form a latticework snowflake of starch, butter and salt.

Once this happens, slide it out of the pan in one motion onto a plate. Then flip, salt lightly again and cook for another 15 to 20 seconds. Then eat! (Alternately, you can flip in a couple pieces with a tin, sturdy spatula.)

Repeat as necessary.

Julia Turshen's Olive Oil-Fried Eggs With Yogurt & Lemon

Ingredients You Need

1/4 cup (60ml) plain yogurt (Greek or not, your choice)

1/2 lemon

Kosher salt

Freshly ground black pepper

2 tablespoons extra-virgin olive oil

2 eggs

1 tablespoon roughly chopped leafy fresh herbs, such as basil, dill, chervil, chives, and/or parsley

How to Make

In a small bowl, combine the yogurt and a big squeeze of juice from the lemon half (don't discard the lemon half) and whisk together. Season to taste with salt and pepper, and adjust the lemon to taste, too. Scrape the mixture onto a plate and spread and swoop it so the yogurt covers most of the plate.

In a nonstick skillet over medium high heat, warm the olive oil. Crack the eggs into the pan and sprinkle each egg with a bit of salt and pepper. Sprinkle a few drops of water (less than a teaspoon) into the skillet, being sure to let the water hit the bottom of the pan and not the eggs, and immediately, carefully cover the pan with a lid or the bottom of another wide, lightweight pan.

Let the eggs cook until the whites are cooked through but the yolks are still a bit wobbly, just a minute or two. Transfer the eggs to the prepared plate, setting them on top of the yogurt, then pour the remaining olive oil from the pan over the top. Squeeze whatever juice remains in the lemon half and scatter over the herbs. Serve immediately.

CHAPTER 4
QUICK AND EASY 80/20 DIET RECIPES
FOR LUNCH

Green Bean and Mushroom Curry

Ingredients You Need

5 tablespoons extra virgiin olive oil

1 yellow onion, cut into half rings

1 piece fresh ginger, peeled and grated

5 garlic cloves, peeled and grated

8 ounces crimini mushrooms, roughly chopped

16 ounces can green beans, drained

1 teaspoon coriander

2 teaspoons cumin

3/4 teaspoon turmeric

3/4 teaspoon garam masala

1/2 teaspoon cayenne pepper

1 teaspoon sea salt

1 tomato, coarsely chopped

How to Make

Place the oil in a large sauté pan and set over medium-high heat.

When the oil is hot, put in the onion. Stir and fry until the onion browns, about 8 minutes.

Add the ginger and garlic. Stir until the garlic starts to brown, 2 to 3 minutes.

Put in the mushrooms, stir, and cook for another 2 minutes.

Add the green beans, coriander, cumin, turmeric, garam masala, cayenne, salt, and tomato.

Lower the heat and let simmer for around 5 minutes. Serve over brown rice.

Vegan Lentil Massaman Curry

Ingredients You Need

80 grams Lentil (uncooked)

20 grams Peanut toasted

260 grams Potatoes – about 2 medium – Peeled quartered and boiled (weight before cook)

50 grams Massaman curry paste

2 teaspoons Brown sugar

1 teaspoon Salt

2 teaspoons Tamarind paste

2 cups Coconut milk

1 cup Water

3 Small onions

How to Make

Let's begin with peeling and cutting the onion. I use small onion so I will just chop them in half. If you use larger onion, you can cut them into quarter pieces.

You can observe by looking at the surface, when it's cracked you will see yellowish oil floating on the top. Now, let fry our curry paste by adding ½ cup of coconut milk into a put, together with the curry paste. Stir the coconut milk and curry paste until the coconut cream is cracked, or when the oil is separate from the milk body.

Add bay leaf and season the curry with sugar, tamarind and salt. Taste the curry and adjust the flavour. The flavour that you are after is salty and follow by a touch of sweet and sour. Next, you can add the rest of the coconut milk and water and then add onion. It will take about 15 minutes for the onion soften. You can let the curry simmer over medium heat. When the onion is cooked, add potatoes, lentil and peanut.

And here it's guys, our lentil Massaman curry! If you like to learn how to cook Thai food, you can join my free work-shop on my website. And if you would like to try my curry paste. I hope you enjoy your curry Will see you next week with awesome recipes and cooking tips have a great day everyone! Sawasdee ka.

Black Garlic and Tarragon Heirloom Tomato

Ingredients You Need

2 pounds heirloom Tomatoes

1 pound nidi linguine

1 1/2 cups frozen sweet corn

1/4 cup black garlic

2 tablespoons butter (plant based or French salted)

2 tablespoons finely chopped tarragon

1 teaspoon fresh cracked pepper

sea salt to taste

How to Make

Chop the tomatoes into small wedges. Finely dice the garlic and tarragon.

Bring a large pot of water to boil (cover the pot with a lid.) When the water begins to boil, add a liberal amount of sea salt. Cook the pasta according to the instructions, checking for an al dente result.

Add the butter and olive oil into a large wide skillet and turn the heat to medium low. When the oils have melted, add in the cracked pepper and whisk until fragrant and the butter is slightly browned.

Now add in the black garlic and whisk quickly until the garlic is well integrated. Next stir in the tarragon.

Add in the tomatoes and stir until incorporated. Allow the tomatoes to reduce for five minutes before adding in the frozen corn, allowing the gravy to cook for another five minutes. Add salt to taste and turn off the heat. The sauce will thicken while the pasta finishes cooking.

Drain the pasta and fold it into the sauce. Garnish with extra virgin olive oil and tarragon. Serve immediately.

Cheesy Roasted Broccoli Potato Soup

Ingredients You Need

8 ounces broccoli florets, preferably fresh

3 cups yukon gold potatoes, peeled and cubed

2 cups baby carrots

1 cup sweet yellow onion (about 1/4 large onion), cubed

2 tablespoons olive oil

salt & pepper

1 tablespoon minced garlic

1 tablespoon diced pimentos, canned

32 ounces vegetable broth

2 cups coconut milk (or other plant milk of choice)

2 cups raw cashews, softened

1/4 cup nutritional yeast

1 teaspoon smoked paprika

1 tablespoon apple cider vinegar

How to Make

Preheat the oven to 425 degrees F. Place the broccoli, potato, carrots, and onion on the same baking sheet and roast in the oven for about 25-30 minutes.

Place 2 cups of cashews in a microwave safe bowl and cover with water. Microwave for 5 minutes to soften them.

While the veggies are roasting, blend together the minced garlic, pimentos, vegetable broth, coconut milk, softened cashews, nutritional yeast, smoked paprika, and apple cider vinegar until smooth and no cashew pieces remain. Pour the soup base into a large pot and heat the soup over medium low heat. Add the roasted vegetables when they are done roasting and continue to heat until the soup thickens. Use an immersion blender and blend until desired soup consistency. If the soup is too thick you can add more milk, broth, or water. If you like a chunkier soup you can pulse to blend the veggies together or you can blend until smooth if you like a smoother soup. If you don't have an immersion blender, you can blend the veggies in your blender and heat. Enjoy the soup right away garnished with leftover roasted broccoli and potato (optional), fresh parsley, microgreens, and hemp seeds!

Salatet Fattoush (California Fattoush Salad) from Reem Assil

Ingredients You Need

Dressing

1 garlic clove, crushed

2 tablespoons tablespoons lemon juice (about 1 lemon)

1 tablespoon pomegranate molasses

1/2 teaspoon kosher salt

1/4 teaspoon freshly ground black pepper

1/4 cup extra-virgin olive oil

Salad

3 cups store-bought pita chips or 2-inch pieces of pita bread, fried

2 cups halved cherry tomatoes

1 Persian cucumber, halved lengthwise and cut into ⅛-inch crescents (about 1 cup)

4 radishes, sliced into thin rounds

1/4 red onion, halved stem to root and thinly sliced into crescents (about 1 cup)

2 cups Little Gem lettuce or chopped Romaine

2 cups loosely packed arugula

Leaves from 2 sprigs of parsley

Leaves from 2 sprigs of mint

1 tablespoon sumac

How to Make

To make the dressing: Combine all of the **Ingredients You Need** in a blender or a bowl and mix or whisk to incorporate. Make sure to whisk well again before using, since the oil will separate.

To assemble the salad: In a medium bowl, toss half the chips with the tomatoes, cucumber, radishes, onion, Little Gem, and 1/4 cup of the dressing.

Lay the arugula on a serving platter and cover evenly with the dressed veggies and chips. Tuck the remaining half of the pita chips into the salad to fill in any gaps. Drizzle the remaining dressing over the salad. Sprinkle the parsley and mint over the dish and top with the sumac.

Classic Miso Eggplant Risotto

Ingredients You Need

1 Eggplant

2-4 tablespoons Olive Oil

8 Scallions

4 Cloves Garlic

1 cup Arborio Rice

1/4 cup White Miso Paste

2 cups Vegetable Broth

1-3 tablespoons Sambal Oelek

2 tablespoons Soy Sauce

1 tablespoon Vegan Butter

1/4 cup Sake

How to Make

Preheat oven to 400°F. Cut the eggplant into half inch pieces. Coat eggplant with 2-3 tbsp olive oil. Roast for 25 - 30 minutes.

Prepare the Risotto: mince the garlic. Dice scallions and reserve 2 tbsp of the green part for a garnish. Heat 1 tbsp of olive oil in a skillet over medium heat. Sauté the garlic and scallions for about 1 minute.

Add Arborio rice, and stir to coat. Cook the rice, stirring often, until it begins to look translucent, about 3-4 minutes.

While the rice is cooking, dissolve white miso paste into 1 1/2 C hot water, and combine with 2 C vegetable broth.Once the rice is shiny and translucent, add the broth 1/2 C at a time. Stir the risotto frequently, adding more broth as the liquid is absorbed. Once all the broth has been absorbed, and the rice is tender and fluffy, remove from heat. (You may run out of broth before the rice reaches this point. This is OK, just use water until the rice is done. OR, if the rice is fluffy before you've used all the broth, that is fine too. Discard what is left).

Stir in the butter. Add sambal oelek to taste; use more if you want a spicier dish. Stir in the sake, if using.

Finish the Eggplant: Once the eggplant has become brown and crispy, remove it from the oven. Transfer to a skillet on low heat. Add the soy sauce and cook until just absorbed.

Assemble the risotto: Divide the risotto into four dishes. Top with roasted eggplant and reserved scallion greens. Top with crispy tofu bites, if desired.

Notes: You can make this meal completely gluten free by subbing in tamari for the soy sauce.

Butternut Squash Spinach Pasta

Ingredients You Need

3-4 cups butternut squash, cubed

2 tablespoons olive oil

1 tablespoon minced garlic

8 ounces gluten-free pasta

1 onion, diced

5 ounces organic spinach

1/2 cup vegetable/no-chicken broth

1/4 cup vegan parmesan cheese

salt, to taste

pepper, to taste

toasted pine nuts, for garnishing

How to Make

Preheat the oven to 400 degrees. Arrange the cubed butternut squash pieces on a baking sheet and drizzle with olive oil and sprinkle with salt and pepper. Roast in the oven until the squash starts to turn golden, about 15-20 minutes.

Meanwhile, cook the pasta according to package directions. In a large skillet, heat 2 tablespoons of olive oil, the minced garlic, and salt over medium heat. Add the diced onion and saute until translucent. Next, add the broth, vegan parmesan cheese, and red pepper flakes. Simmer over low heat to combine the flavors.

Drain the pasta, then add it to the skillet. Finally add the butternut squash and spinach to the skillet, cooking for a few more minutes until the spinach begins to wilt. Serve with more vegan parmesan cheese, toasted pine nuts and red pepper flakes if desired!

Grilled peach and watercress salad

Ingredients You Need

4 cups watercress, or arugula

2 peaches

1/4 cup crumbled feta, or blue cheese

1/4 cup toasted walnuts, or pine nuts

1 tablespoon balsamic vinegar

1 tablespoon pomegranate molasses

1 tablespoon olive oil

How to Make

The salad is very easy to put together. We just need to grill the peaches. Just cut the peach in half, discard the pit and place them on hot grill. It takes about 8-10 minutes to get nice grill marks and caramelize the peaches. Put them aside and let them chill.

Next mix pomegranate molasses and balsamic together. If you have a good quality balsamic reduction that is thick, you can use it, as it's sweet and has that tang that we need for the salad. Add olive oil and mix well.

Now that we have our grilled peaches cooled down, cut them into bite size pieces. Build the salad: place the salad leaves on the plate, add feta, peaches, walnuts, drizzle the dressing and that's it, simple, beautiful and delicious.

Cheesy Orzo with Roasted Cherry Tomatoes

Ingredients You Need

300 grams /10.6 oz orzo

400 grams /14.1 oz cherry tomatoes

70 grams /2.5 oz grated Parmesan

1.5 cups vegetable broth

1 cup whole milk

4 garlic cloves, minced

1 shallot, finely chopped

4 tablespoons olive oil

4 tablespoons pine nuts

4 thyme sprigs

salt + black pepper, to taste

crushed red pepper flakes, for serving

flaky salt, for serving

How to Make

Preheat the oven to 200°C/400°F.

Place the cherry tomatoes in a baking sheet, sprinkle with 2 tbsp olive oil. Season with a pinch of salt and black pepper. Slide into the oven for 15 minutes.

Meanwhile, heat a large non-stick skillet or Dutch oven over high heat. Add pine nuts and toast until golden, about 1 minute. Remove from skillet.

Make the orzo. Lower the heat, add the remaining oil, garlic and shallot, cook until soft, about 1 minute.

Add orzo, stir until fragrant, about 1 minute. Pour in vegetable broth and milk. Bring to a boil, cover and reduce the heat to a simmer. Cook, stirring occasionally, until the liquid is absorbed, about 10-15 minutes or according to package instructions. Add a splash of water if the orzo looks too dry.

Stir in Parmesan. Taste, and adjust salt and black pepper.

Top with roasted cherry tomatoes and their released juices. Sprinkle with flaky salt and red pepper flakes. Serve with toasted pine nuts, enjoy!

Yaki Udon- Stir-fried Udon Noodles With Vegetables

Ingredients You Need

2 tablespoons Cooking Oil

600 grams Udon Noodles(Cooked)

320 grams Cabbage

110 grams Carrot

10 pieces Dried Shiitake Mushroom

60 grams Brown Onion

8 grams Crushed Garlic

3 tablespoons Light Soy Sauce

2 tablespoons Dark Soy Sauce

2 tablespoons Vegan Oyster Sauce

4 tablespoons Black Vinegar

2 tablespoons Mirin

2 teaspoons Sesame Oi

1/4 teaspoon Ground White Pepper

4 tablespoons Mushroom Soaking Water

2 tablespoons (Garnish) Black and White Sesame seeds

1 handful (Garnish) Shredded Nori

1 handful (Garnish) Sliced Spring Onion

How to Make

Firstly, we gonna soak Shiitake mushrooms in hot boiling water for 15 minutes, then slice them.

Meanwhile, we slice the cabbage, carrot, and brown onion, also finely chop the garlic.

Cook packed udon noodles in the pot with boiling water for 1-2 minutes until the noodles are loose. Drain them then set them aside.

Heat up the frying pan with oil on medium-high heat, saute brown onion, Shiitake mushroom, carrot, and garlic until they are softened.

Add cabbage to the pan and mushroom soaking liquid. Cook until cabbage is softened. Then add light and dark soy sauce, oyster sauce, and ground white pepper in, cook for 1-2 minutes.

Return udon noodles back to the pan, stir and mix with the sauces until noodles are well coated.

Add black vinegar in, stir and cook for further minutes. Taste to see if more salt is needed.

Finish with sesame oil, then garnish with black and white sesame seeds, shredded Nori, and spring onion.

Air Fryer Buffalo Cauliflower Tacos

Ingredients You Need

Bean purée & Greek yogurt dressing

1 can canellini beans

1/4 onion minced

3 pieces garlic minced

1 teaspoon french dried thyme

1/2 teaspoon onion powder

1 teaspoon garlic powder

1/2 lemon juice divided in 2 parts

Salt and pepper to taste

1 kirby cucumber

1 tablespoon butter (unsalted)

1/2 cup vegetable broth

1 cup greek plain yogurt

Buffalo Cauliflower

1 large cauliflower head chopped

1 teaspoon salt

fresh cracked pepper

2 tablespoons melted butter

2 pieces garlic minced

3/4 cup Franks hot sauce original

1 teaspoon garlic powder

2 tablespoons olive oil

Flour tortillas

How to Make

Bean purée & Greek yogurt dressing

Sauté over medium heat, onions and garlic until they are light brown, add canelli beans and mash them with a potato masher. Add broth, one part of the lemon juice, french dried thyme. Mix and let simmer until broth has been absorbed, adjust salt and pepper to taste.

Chop cucumber in small pieces, mix in with yogurt, one other part of lemon juice and add onion and garlic powders. Adjust salt.

Buffalo Cauliflower

Chopped cauliflower in medium pieces, toss in a bowl with salt, pepper and garlic powder and olive oil. Place it in the Air Fryer at 390 for 20-40 min, pause it from time to time and toss around to make sure it gets evely "fried".

Melt butter in the microwave, add minced galirc, onion powder, and buffalo sauce. Pour over the fried cauliflower and mix.

Serve now: Heat up flour tortillas, spread the bean purée, add buffalo cauliflower, your favorite greens and the greek yougurt sauce. Enjoy!

Kale & Acorn Squash Cornbread Panzanella

Ingredients You Need

Salad **Ingredients You Need**

1 acorn squash

1 bunch lacinato kale

3 cups cornbread (cubed)

2 bartlett pears (red ones if you can find)

1 pomegranate (seeded)

1 shallot

2 teaspoons macadamia nut oil

3 tablespoons maple syrup (divided)

3-4 sage leaves

Dressing **Ingredients You Need**

2 tablespoons maple syrup

2 tablespoons apple cider vinegar

1/3 cup macadamia nut oil

2 teaspoons dijon mustard

1 teaspoon salt (to taste)

1 teaspoon pepper

1/2 teaspoon sage leaves (finely chopped)

How to Make

Cube your cornbread and time permitting let it sit out for several hours to firm up a bit.

Drizzle 2 tablespoons of maple syrup and your chopped sage leaves on the cubes and toss lightly.

Roast the croutons 10-15 mins until crispy and golden turning once during cooking.

Lower your oven temp to 375 degrees and line a sheet pan with parchment paper.

Microwave your acorn squash for approx 3 mins and remove and cut the ends off, seed the squash and place cut side down on a cutting board and cut into slices. Place the slices on the parchment lined sheet pan and brush both sides with approx. 1 tablespoon of your maple syrup.

Roast for 30 mins or until tender flipping once in between cooking, set aside.

Finely slice your shallot and add it to a small microwave safe dish with the mac nut oil, microwave 1 min at a time turning the shallots in the dish until they become crispy. (should take a bout 3 mins).

Make your dressing by whisking all ingredients together in a small bowl or glass Pyrex measuring cup.

Wash and de-rib your kale and tear into bite sized pieces and add to your salad bowl, add your croutons, top with sliced red bartlett pears, pomegranate seeds, and roasted acorn squash and crispy shallots. Toss with dressing and enjoy!

Quinoa Salad with Seasonal Vegetables and Fresh Lemon Dressing

Ingredients:

- 1 cup cooked and cooled quinoa

- 1 cup seasonal vegetables (chopped tomatoes, sliced cucumber, shredded carrots)

- 1/2 cup fresh chopped mint

- 1/4 cup pomegranate seeds for garnish

For Lemon Dressing:

- 3 tablespoons olive oil

- Juice of one lemon

- 1 teaspoon honey

- Salt and pepper to taste

Instructions:

1. In a large bowl, mix quinoa, seasonal vegetables, and mint.

2. In a small bowl, whisk together the lemon dressing ingredients thoroughly.

3. Pour the lemon dressing over the salad and gently toss until all ingredients are coated with the dressing.

4. Serve the salad in a serving dish and sprinkle pomegranate seeds on top for a burst of color and flavor.

Palak daal

Ingredients You Need

1 cup dry white urad daal, soaked for at least 3 hours

6 cups water

1/2 pound fresh spinach, chopped

1 tablespoon fresh ginger, peeled and minced

1/2 teaspoon turmeric powder

1 serrano pepper, minced

2 medium tomatoes, chopped

1/2 teaspoon sea salt

2 tablespoons coconut oil

1/2 teaspoon cumin seeds

1/4 teaspoon cayenne pepper

1/8 teaspoon asafetida

2 teaspoons lemon juice

How to Make

Soak the urad daal in cool filtered water, for at least two hours but preferably overnight. Rinse well, until the water runs clear.

Combine the soaked daal and 6 cups water in a large pot over medium heat. Bring to a boil. Then add the ginger and turmeric, spinach, tomatoes, and serrano pepper.

Reduce heat to a simmer, cover, let cook about 2 hours or until the lentils are very soft. I tend to add a small amount of water half way through. Add the salt.

In a separate pan, melt the coconut oil and add the cumin seeds. Cook over medium heat until the seeds pop. Add the cayenne pepper and asafetida, cook briefly until fragrant. Be careful not to burn the spices.

Add the oil & spice mixture to the pot and cook for another 4-5 minutes, stirring to combine. Then add the lemon.

Serve with a spoonful brown rice to balance the spice, some fresh cilantro. Also good with a dollop of plain coconut yogurt.

Turmeric Dry Tofu Curry

Ingredients You Need

For the paste

180 grams whole shallot (150g peeled)

dutch red chilli - deseed for less heat

25 grams peeled garlic (4 cloves)

30 grams turmeric, fresh - washed (I don't peel)

4 lemongrass, woody ends triimmed, and outer layer removed, and sliced

5 kaffir lime, destemed

1.5 teaspoons 1.5 tsp white pepper

35 grams oil - I used rapeseed

.5 teaspoons salt

For the curry

300 grams red rice

600 grams water

.5 teaspoons salt

3 kaffir lime, whole

1 lemongrass, bruised- - lightly crushing the end, using the back of the knife or a rolling pin

1 tablespoon coconut oil

rapeseed or coconut oil

1 portion curry paste

1 tablespoon coconut sugar

600 grams firm tofu

50 grams cornflour

1 teaspoon salt

1.5 teaspoons turmeric

.5 teaspoons white pepper

300 grams sprouting broccoli, cut into ½ cm pieces

4 kaffir lime leaves, destemmed and finely sliced

20 grams juice lime (1/2 - 1 lime)

40 grams coriander

20 grams thai basil

How to Make

For the fragrant rice. Rinse the rice well with fresh water. Place in a medium pan with a lid, along with the lemongrass, kaffir lime, coconut oil salt and water. Cover, bring to the boil, turn down, and steam for 30 minutes. Once it's ready, turn off the heat and leave the lid on for a further 10 minutes.

Prepare and blend spice paste ingredients, in a blender blend until smooth.

In a wide-based pan, on medium heat, heat the pan, add 30g or (3 tablespoons) of the oil to the pan, then add the curry paste, cook for 15 minutes, stirring every few minutes to stop it sticking and so it cooks evenly. Add the sugar and cook for another 5 minutes until darkened. Remove the paste from the pan, clean the pan and prepare the tofu.

Cut the tofu into inch pieces cubes. Mix the corn flour, turmeric, white pepper and salt medium bowl. Heat the pan on medium heat, and add the remaining oil. Shake the tofu in the mixing bowl to coat in the cornflour turmeric mix. When the pan is hot, using tongs shake off any excessive flour and cook the tofu pieces, turning to crispen all sides of the tofu. You may need to do this in batches if your pan isn't big enough to fit them without overcrowding. When they're ready, remove and place on a plate lined with kitchen roll to drain excess oil.

Add the broccoli to the pan, with a splash of water, cook for 3-4 minutes, until tender. Add the paste back in, with a splash of water to loosen if needed then add the tofu and kaffir lime, mix well and heat through. Finish with the fresh lime, coriander and Thai basil, if using.

Serve with your fragrant rice.

Creamy One Pot Lemon Pasta

Ingredients You Need

1 lemon, zest and juice

12 ounces fettuccine

1/2 cup heavy cream

1/2 cup grated parmesan

1 cup reserved pasta water

1/2 teaspoon kosher salt

black pepper, to taste

fresh parsley, for topping

How to Make

Bring a large pot of salted water to a boil. Cook your pasta according to package instructions. Right before it is done, save a cup of the pasta water. Then drain and set aside.

Add cream and lemon zest to the same pot over medium-low heat. Let it simmer for about 2-3 minutes until it thickens slightly.

Add in your cooked pasta to the cream sauce. Slowly add in the parmesan and most of the pasta water. Tossing constantly, you want the parmesan to melt as you add it in. Add in more pasta water to thin out the pasta sauce as needed (You might not need all of it).

Add in 1 tbsp of lemon juice and salt. Taste for and adjust for seasoning.

Serve and top with additional parmesan, parsley, and black pepper.

Corn Ribs

Ingredients You Need

4 large ears of corn

2 tablespoons olive oil

1 tablespoon smoked paprika

1 teaspoon garlic powder

1 teaspoon onion powder

2 tablespoons BBQ sauce

chopped cilantro

cojita cheese / queso fresco

How to Make

Preheat the oven to 400°F (200°C). Shuck the corn and carefully cut each ear into "ribs" by slicing vertically between the rows of kernels.

In a bowl, toss the corn ribs with olive oil, smoked paprika, garlic powder, onion powder, chili powder, salt, and black pepper. Ensure the corn ribs are evenly coated with the seasonings.

Place the seasoned corn ribs on a baking sheet lined with parchment paper, making sure they are in a single layer.

Roast the corn ribs in the preheated oven for 20-25 minutes or until they are golden brown and slightly crispy, turning them halfway through for even cooking.

Remove the corn ribs from the oven and transfer them to a serving plate. Sprinkle with chopped fresh parsley or cilantro for a burst of freshness. Add as much cheese as you want! I love queso fresco for this recipe! Serve the corn ribs hot with lime wedges on the side for squeezing over the top. Optional: add queso fresco on top!

Delicious Corn Ribs with Queso Fresco

Ingredients You Need

4 large ears of corn

2 tablespoons olive oil

1 tablespoon smoked paprika

1 teaspoon garlic powder

1 teaspoon onion powder

2 tablespoons BBQ sauce

chopped cilantro

cojita cheese / queso fresco

How to Make

Preheat the oven to 400°F (200°C). Shuck the corn and carefully cut each ear into "ribs" by slicing vertically between the rows of kernels.

In a bowl, toss the corn ribs with olive oil, smoked paprika, garlic powder, onion powder, chili powder, salt, and black pepper. Ensure the corn ribs are evenly coated with the seasonings.

Place the seasoned corn ribs on a baking sheet lined with parchment paper, making sure they are in a single layer.

Roast the corn ribs in the preheated oven for 20-25 minutes or until they are golden brown and slightly crispy, turning them halfway through for even cooking.

Remove the corn ribs from the oven and transfer them to a serving plate. Sprinkle with chopped fresh parsley or cilantro for a burst of freshness. Add as much cheese as you want! I love queso fresco for this recipe! Serve the corn ribs hot with lime wedges on the side for squeezing over the top. Optional: add queso fresco on top!

Classic Parsely Bowl

Ingredients You Need

One large red capsicum deseeded and shredded

One large brown onion shredded

Three garlic cloves peeled and minced

One tsp of salt

A pinch of black crushed pepper

One tsp of paprika

Two tbsps of cold pressed extra virgin olive oil

A pinch of chopped parsley for garnish

How to Make

Heat a medium sized pan at medium heat with oil and throw in the onions once the oil is heated and cook for 2 minutes or until the onions become brown. Next throw in all the ingredients in the pan and cook for 8 minutes or until everything is well cooked.

Once all the ingredients are well cooked turn off the stove and let everything cool. Next with a food processor pour in the cooked vegetables and process them for 30 seconds to a minute or until the consistency becomes slightly pasty and chunky.

Pour the dip into a nice lovely bowl with parsley on top and enjoy!

Summer Corn Pizza

Ingredients You Need

Your favorite pizza dough recipe

4 teaspoons extra virgin olive oil

2 garlic cloves, crushed

1 medium yellow onion, sliced

1 red bell pepper, sliced

1 yellow bell pepper, sliced

2 ears of corn

1 tablespoon cornmeal

1 cup mozzarella cheese, shredded

1 teaspoon kosher salt

1-2 teaspoons crushed red pepper

How to Make

Preheat oven to 500.

Heat a small skillet over medium heat. Add olive oil and garlic to pan. Cook 2 minutes or until fragrant, be careful not to brown. Remove oil from pan and discard garlic. Add a swirl of oil to pan and add onions and bell peppers. Sauté till soft, about 5 minutes. Set aside. Cut corn from cob and add to vegetables.

Lightly flour surface. Sprinkle with about 1 tablespoon of cornmeal. Roll out pizza dough into a 13 inch circle. Transfer to a baking sheet. Brush dough with garlic oil. Top with vegetable mixture. Cover with shredded cheese, salt, and red pepper.

Bake for 15 minutes or until golden brown. Slice and serve.

Beet Pizza

Ingredients You Need

Pizza Dough (enough for two 10" pies)

2 1/2 cups all-purpose flour, about 11.25 oz., or 319 grams; I use King Arthur all-purpose unbleached flour

1 1/2 teaspoons kosher salt, about 5 grams

3/4 teaspoon active dry yeast, not rapid rise, about 3 grams

8 ounces lukewarm water, about 227 grams

1/4 cup olive oil, about 50 grams

Beet Pizza (double the quantities for a second pie)

Pizza dough, about 10 ounces

1 large beet, trimmed with 2" of tops attached, roasted in foil, peeled and sliced about 1/8" thick

1/4 to 1/2 cup whole milk ricotta cheese

2 ounces goat cheese

1/4 cup red onion, sliced very thin

1 sprig fresh thyme

olive oil

kosher salt and fresh cracked black pepper

How to Make

Pizza Dough (enough for two 10" pies)

These instructions are for a stand mixer, but you can do it all by hand, if you so choose. In the bowl of a stand mixer fitted with the paddle attachment, mix flour and salt together.

Dissolve yeast into warm water. Stir in the oil. With mixer on low speed, pour the liquid into the flour until dough comes together.

Scrape off the paddle and switch to the dough hook. Knead for 5 or so minutes.

Scrape mixer bowl and hook, and gather dough into a ball. Place in a well-oiled bowl. Cover bowl tightly with plastic wrap, lay a dish towel over it and place in a warm spot, like in the microwave. Sometimes, before putting the dough in, I heat a mug-full of water, to get the microwave nice and warm.

Let rise for 1 hour. Punch dough down, and let rise for another hour.

This step is totally optional, but worth it if you have all day. Punch dough down again and let rise for 2 - 3 more hours. Alternatively, you can stash the dough in the fridge overnight after the first rise. Bring refrigerated dough to room temperature about an hour before forming pizzas.

Divide dough into two equal pieces, 10 ounces each (roughly 284 grams), weighing it with a kitchen scale if you have one. On a lightly floured board, gently form into a round ball by folding the dough top and bottom, then left and right, like an envelope. Set the dough balls aside, seam sides down, on a lightly floured pan. If you're only making one pie, place the second dough ball in a freezer bag and freeze.

Beet Pizza (double the quantities for a second pie)

Place a pizza stone on bottom-most rack in oven. Preheat oven to BROIL, at highest heat, at least a half hour before you will bake the pizza.

Divide dough into two equal pieces, 10 ounces each (roughly 284 grams), weighing it with a kitchen scale if you have one. On a lightly floured board, gently form into a round ball by folding the dough top and bottom, then left and right, like an envelope. Set the dough balls aside, seam sides down, on a lightly floured pan. If you're only making one pie, place the second dough ball in a freezer bag and freeze.

Lightly flour a quarter-sheet pan (9" x 12"), or a 12" pizza pan, cover with parchment paper, and lightly sprinkle some flour in the parchment paper.

Flatten dough very slightly, and fold in top, bottom, left side, right side, towards center. Turn over, and gently form into a round. Place on lightly floured parchment-lined sheet pan, sprinkle with flour and cover with a kitchen towel. Let rest 10 minutes.

Place ball of dough on a very lightly-oiled (just a dab to keep the paper in place) parchment-lined 12" pizza pan. Dust dough lightly with flour and press down with your fingertips as you turn the pie and spread the dough evenly in all **How to Make**until you have a nice thin layer, about 1/4" thick. It probably won't cover the entire pan; that's okay. If dough is not cooperating, it helps to let the dough rest for a few minutes.

Spread ricotta onto pizza dough with a small offset spatula if you have one, leaving about a ½ inch border. Or dollop the ricotta on top willynilly, however you like. Scatter the beet slices in a single layer over the ricotta. You might not need to use the whole beet. If you want, place some of the roasted stem ends on top, too. Next, shower your red onion slices over the top. Then, spoon little nuggets of goat cheese over. Strip the thyme leaves off of the sprig and sprinkle over the pizza. Lastly, just a touch of salt and pepper, a drizzle of olive oil, and your pizza is ready to bake!

Place pan directly on pizza stone. Or, if you've got a pizza peel, pull the parchment and pizza onto the peel, then slide parchment and pizza directly onto pizza stone. Turn heat to 550 degrees F. Bake for 5 minutes, or until crust is nicely browned and crisp, and bottom of pizza has some nicely browned spots as well. Use a long-handled metal spatula or metal tongs, or the pizza peel, to lift up the pizza and take a peek underneath. The parchment will turn black, but it won't catch fire, so don't worry.

Alternatively, if you've got a pizza peel, pull the parchment and pizza onto the peel, then slide parchment and pizza directly onto pizza stone. Bake for 5 to 8 minutes or until crust is nicely browned and crisp , and pizza has some nicely browned spots as well. Use a long-handled metal spatula, or the pizza peel, to lift up the pizza and take a peek underneath. Cheese should be bubbly, and the bottom crust should have some brown spots.

Remove from oven, add a touch more salt or oil if desired, cut into pieces and enjoy!

Repeat with the second ball of pizza dough.

Mint and Green Pea Risotto, with Roasted Tomatoes

Ingredients You Need

The Risotto

2 tablespoons Extra virgin olive oil

1 white onion, finely chopped

2 Garlic cloves, crushed

2 cups Risotto rice

1 1/2 cups white wine

6-7 cups vegetable stock

1 large bunches Fresh Mint, finely chopped

2 1/2 cups frozen peas

The Tomatoes

4 Large tomatoes, halved

a couple pinches Salt, pepper and sugar

3 tablespoons extra virgin olive oil

How to Make

Heat the oven to 160C. Place the halved tomatoes cut side up with the olive oil and seasoning on top, and put in the oven. Keep an eye on them whilst you are making the risotto, they take around 20-30 minutes to cook.

Meanwhile, Sautee the onion and garlic in the olive oil in a large sauteeing pan for 5 minutes, or until soft. Add risotto rice, and stir to coat for about 1 minute. Add white wine and cook for a further 4 minutes. Gradually add the stock and continuously stir for 10-15 minutes, or until the risotto is thick and the rice is "al dente".

Meanwhile, put half the peas into a bowl and pour some boiling water over them (just until they go soft). Drain and then puree until fairly smooth in a food processor/blender. Set aside.

About 5 minutes towards the end of the cooking time, add the pureed peas, the other frozen peas, fresh mint, and stir in. Once the risotto is ready, serve with the hot roasted tomatoes on top, and some extra mint leaves for garnish!

Syrian Lemony Red Lentil Soup with Coriander, Cumin & Garlic (Addes Soup)

Ingredients You Need

1 1/2 cups red lentils

6 cups water

4 cloves garlic crushed

2 teaspoons coriander

1 teaspoon salt

1 teaspoon cumin

1 1/4 tablespoons olive oil

juice of 1-2 lemons

1 tablespoon flour

2 tablespoons water

How to Make

Rinse the lentils, then put in a pot with the water and bring to a boil. Cook the lentils for about 45 minutes on medium fire till they become thick and creamy. Squeeze the lemon into the pot and cook 10 -15 minutes longer

In a small bowl mix the garlic, coriander, cumin and salt till it forms a paste. Put the olive oil in a small frying pan and add the paste and saute till golden for 2-3 minutes. Add to the hot soup and let cook another 10 minutes.

Mix the flour with the water and using a strainer, strain into the soup, stirring the soup constantly, so there are no lumps. Cook another 2-3 minutes. Garnish with sprigs of cilantro or parsley

Corn Chowder (vegan)

Ingredients You Need

2 quarts vegetable stock

4 waxy white potatoes

4 large cloves garlic

1 large yellow onion

1 cups coconut milk

2 lbs. frozen corn

1 handful fresh thyme leaves

2 tablespoons extra virgin olive oil

1 teaspoon cumin

1 tablespoon Sriracha hot sauce

1 teaspoon turmeric

3 tablespoons flour

Salt

pepper

Fresh flat-leaf parsley (for garnish)

How to Make

Take the corn out of the freezer and put it on the counter to begin thawing out. Heat the olive oil in a large soup pot over medium-low heat. Chop up the onion and garlic and add it to the soup pot. Sauté for about 10 minutes until the veggies are soft, stirring frequently. Remove the thyme from the stems and add the leaves to the onions and garlic. Add the turmeric, cumin, and Sriracha. Stir well and sauté for another minute. Add the flour and stir well. Pour in all the vegetable stock and bring the soup up to a boil. Chop the potatoes into cubes and add them to the soup. Pour in the coconut milk, stir, and boil for about 5-10 more minutes. Add the corn to the soup (it's okay if it's not completely defrosted), stir, and cover with a lid. Simmer for 20 minutes. Chop up fresh parsley and sprinkle it into bowls of the soup when you're ready to serve. Tip 1: I like using organic frozen corn because it cuts down on my preparation time and really retains its crunchiness. Use fresh corn if you're up to it, but I think frozen corn is easiest. Tip 2: I think one tablespoon of Sriracha gives this the perfect amount of heat, but if you're sensitive to spicy foods, I recommend using just a dash at a time and taste testing to make sure you don't over spice it to your liking.

Miami Salad

Ingredients You Need

Dressing

1 teaspoon Dijon mustard

1/2 teaspoon molasses

3 fresh limes (5 tablespoons of juice, 1½ teaspoons zest)

1 teaspoon white wine vinegar

2 cloves garlic, grated

1 teaspoon kosher salt

1/2 teaspoon freshly ground black pepper

1/2 cup olive oil (plus 2 tablespoons)

Salad

4 cups baby romaine lettuce

3 cups baby spinach

3 ears corn, kernels removed

1 red bell pepper, cut into 1-by-½-inch pieces,stems, ribs and seeds discarded

3 scallions, trimmed and cut into 1-by-½-inch pieces, root ends discarded

1/2 cup sliced black olives

1 (14-ounce) can hearts of palm, drained and rinsed

1 (9-ounce) jar artichoke hearts (not marinated) or frozen artichokes

2 microwaved, baked, or boiled sweet potatoes, at room temperature, peeled and cut into 2-inch cubes

2 medium dill pickles, cut into 1/2-inch dice

3 avocados

How to Make

Prepare the dressing by combining the Dijon mustard, molasses, lime juice and zest, vinegar, garlic, salt, and pepper in a mixing bowl and whisk to blend thoroughly. While whisking, drizzle in the oil until the mixture is thoroughly blended and emulsified. Set aside.

Combine the romaine lettuce, spinach, corn kernels, red pepper, scallions, olives, hearts of palm, artichokes, sweet potatoes, pickles into a large serving bowl. Cut the avocados into 2-inch cubes.

Whisk the dressing once more to blend and pour it over the salad. Toss gently to coat and serve.

Colorful Salad with Orange Vinaigrette

Ingredients You Need

3 pieces Pink radish

1/4 piece Beetroot

1 Lettuce

8-10 Mint leaves

2 tablespoons Crushed nuts such as peanuts

1 Orange

1/4 cup Olive oil

1 teaspoon Balsalmic vinegar

Salt and pepper to taste

How to Make

Shred, cut and tear vegetables. Chop nuts and pick out mint leaves.

Section orange and squeeze out the juice into a bowl. Add balsamic vinegar and season with salt and pepper.

Whisk and add olive oil to emulsify. Drizzle vinaigrette over vegetables and garnish with chopped nuts.

Kimchi Grilled Cheese

Ingredients You Need

2 slices sandwich bread (I used wheat)

1 tablespoon butter, enough to thinly butter one side of each slice

2 slices American cheese (but any meltable kind will work well pepperjack, cheddar, Colby, provolone are just a few that come to mind! And of course you can always add more cheese.)

about 1/3 cups kimchi, drained, patted dry, and chopped (enough for one or two layers)

How to Make

Butter one side of each slice of bread, taking care to spread the butter to the very edges. Note:

Alternatively, you can melt the butter directly into the skillet and then fry the bread in it, which I do not do. I find buttering the slices themselves to be a more precise use of the amount of butter I'll need, and is likely a lesser amount as well. Also, if I have a toaster handy I like to lightly toast my bread beforehand, but that's totally optional.

Heat a skillet over medium heat, then place the slices of bread butter-side down. Next, you'll need to add one slice of cheese to each slice of bread. If you're using cheese that takes a bit of time to melt, you may want to add your slices right away. If you're using regular processed Kraft, then wait until the bread is lightly browned underneath before adding the cheese.

Layer kimchi over one slice only — this makes flipping the other one to combine them easier.

Optionally, you can panfry the kimchi on its own to get it warmed up and add some crispy bits, as well as avoid sogginess. If you're feeling really decadent you can panfry the kimchi in butter.

Let the bread fry on the skillet until golden brown and the cheese is melted on top. Depending on your skillet, you may want to lower the heat at this point to medium-low or low heat to prevent burning. Finally, flip the cheese-only slice onto the kimchi-and-cheese slice (highly technical terms are these) to complete the sandwich, and press lightly on top with a spatula to get them to really squish together. Remove and let cool, then slice and serve!

Roasted Cauliflower and Garlic Pizza

Ingredients You Need

1 head cauliflower, florets separated and thinly sliced

Olive oil

Kosher salt and ground black pepper, to taste

1 head garlic, top of bulb trimmed off until tops of cloves are exposed

Nonstick cooking spray and/or cornmeal, for pan

1 ball of pizza dough, store-bought or homemade

1/2 cup cream cheese

2 Roma tomatoes, sliced into 1/4-inch thick slices

1/4 cup shredded Parmesan cheese

1-1/2 tablespoons chopped fresh chives

How to Make

Preheat oven to 400°. Place cauliflower on rimmed baking pan. Drizzle with oil and sprinkle with salt and pepper. Place garlic on piece of foil; drizzle with a small amount of oil and tightly wrap foil around bulb. Place garlic on same pan as cauliflower. Roast cauliflower until very brown, about 50 minutes, stirring occasionally. Transfer cauliflower to bowl, then return pan with garlic to oven. Roast garlic until it is dark golden brown and very soft, about 10 minutes longer. Let garlic stand for 5 minutes or until cool enough to touch.

Increase oven to 450°. Press pizza dough into large circle on pizza stone or pan (spray with cooking spray or sprinkle with cornmeal first if you're worried about dough sticking). Bake 10 minutes or until light golden brown and almost cooked through.

Meanwhile, squeeze garlic from it's cloves into a small bowl. Add cream cheese and mash together with a fork.

Remove crust from oven. Spread with cream cheese mixture, then top with cauliflower, tomatoes, cheese and chives. Bake 5 to 7 minutes longer, or until crust is cooked through and toppings are hot.

CHAPTER 6
QUICK AND EASY 80/20 DIET RECIPES
FOR 20 INDULGENCE DAY

Sweet Potato Roll with Cream Cheese Filling

Ingredients You Need

For the filling

8 ounces cream cheese, softened

4 tablespoons butter, softened

1 cup powdered sugar, sifted

1 teaspoon vanilla extract

For the rolled cake

4 eggs

1 cup sugar

2/3 cup baked sweet potato pulp, mashed with fork

3/4 cup cake flour

1 teaspoon baking powder

2 teaspoons cinnamon

1/2 teaspoon salt

How to Make

To make filling: Beat together cream cheese and butter. Stir in sifted powdered sugar and vanilla extract. Continue stirring until smooth. Set filling aside.

To make rolled cake: Beat together eggs and sugar with the whisk attachment of a stand mixer. Add sweet potato to mixture until it has the consistency of a foam cake, about 10 minutes.

In another bowl, sift together cake flour, baking powder, cinnamon, and salt.

Fold in dry ingredients to wet ingredients, stirring until combined.

Spread batter onto 10x15-inch jelly roll pan lined with parchment paper. Bake at 375°F for 15 minutes. Allow to cool for 15 minutes.

Remove parchment paper and place cake on clean tea towel without any iron-on type designs inside jelly roll pan. Bake an additional 10 minutes. Roll cake up in towel from 10-inch side. Cool the cake for 20 minutes.

Unroll cake and place on plastic wrap. Evenly spread filling over cake. Roll tightly andand cover with plastic wrap. Chill 2 hours prior to serving.

Carrot-Halwa Blondie Bars (Carrot Cake Blondies)

Ingredients You Need

2 cups all-purpose flour

3 teaspoons double acting baking powder (leveled)

2 cups shredded carrots

1/2 cup whole milk

5 tablespoons sugar

1/2 cup raisins

one 14-ounce can condensed milk

8 tablespoons unsalted butter, melted

5 to 7 pods cardamom seeds, crushed

1/8 teaspoon ground nutmeg

1/2 cup slivered almonds

How to Make

Preheat oven to 350° F.

In a large bowl, sieve together the flour and baking powder. Set aside.

Combine the shredded carrots, whole milk, sugar, and raisins in an oven proof bowl. Pour the condensed milk over top.

Mix well and microwave for 5 to 8 minutes, until the carrots are soft and have lost their raw taste.

Add the melted butter, cardamom, and nutmeg. Combine well. (I prefer to add the spices after the carrots are cooked to ensure that the essential oils in the spices do not dissipate)

Pour the carrot mixture into the center of the mixing bowl containing the flour. Fold it in gently from the sides towards the center. Take care not to over-mix, as this can cause the gluten to bind together, resulting in a tough and leathery texture.

Spread evenly onto a sheet tray and sprinkle with slivered almonds. Bake for 20 to 25 minutes, or until the top is golden-brown.

Allow to cool, cut into squares, and serve. These bars freeze well and will keep for up to a month in the freezer.

Perfect Hot Chocolate

Ingredients You Need

1 ounce semisweet or dark chocolate

1 tablespoon unsweetened cocoa powder

1 cup milk

2 tablespoons granulated sugar (optional, to taste)

1 pinch salt

How to Make

In a small saucepan, mix the chocolate, cocoa powder and 1/2 cup of the milk over low heat. Stir continuously until the chocolate is completely melted.

Add the rest of the milk and the salt. Stir, then allow to heat the rest of the way through.

Stir in sugar to taste. Pour into a mug and top with marshmallows or whipped cream, if desired.

Mom's Flapjacks

Ingredients You Need

1 cup butter

2/3 cup sugar

heaped 1/3 cups golden syrup

4 1/4 cups 1 minute oats

1 heaping tablespoons flour

1 pinch salt

2 handfuls pumpkin seeds

1/4 cup sunflower seeds

scant 1/4 cups sesame seeds

How to Make

Heat the oven to 350F/180C/Gas 4. If you have a fan or convection oven reduce the temperature and cooking time but ideally turn the fan off. Line a 20 x 30 cm baking tin with greaseproof paper (parchment paper)

In a large pan, heat together the butter, sugar and golden syrup over a gentle heat, stirring until the butter has melted. Tip in the flour, oats, salt and seeds and stir to combine.

Tip your pan and spread evenly without pressing down too hard. Bake in the oven for roughly 20-25 minutes or until lightly golden (they will be slightly darker at the edges). Cut them, whilst still in the pan, straight from the oven and then leave to cool and set in the pan.

Brown Butter and Butternut Loaf

Ingredients You Need

For the butternut loaf:

1 cup unsalted butter

3 large eggs

1 1/2 cups sugar

1/2 cup packed light brown sugar

2 cups puréed roasted butternut squash

3 cups all purpose flour

1 teaspoon salt

2 teaspoons baking powder

2 teaspoons baking soda

1/2 teaspoon ground nutmeg (preferrably freshly ground)

For the brown butter icing.

5 tablespoons salted butter

1 1/2 cups confectioners sugar, plus more if needed

1 teaspoon vanilla extract

How to Make

For the butternut loaf:

Preheat your oven to 350° F, and grease two 9-inch loaf pans.

In a large frying pan, heat the butter over medium high heat. It will melt first, and then start to foam. Turn the heat down to medium. Stir the melted butter almost constantly, scraping any browning bits from the bottom of the pan. When the butter has turned a brown color and smells rich and nutty, remove it from the heat. (This should take about 7 minutes). Allow it to cool for about 10 minutes.

In the bowl of a standing mixer, beat together the eggs and sugars on high speed for several minutes, until the color has lightened (Random side note: in Norwegian this is called an "eggedosis"). Scrape in the browned butter and beat for another couple of minutes, until the mixture is smooth.

Add the puréed squash to the wet ingredients and beat until smooth and uniformly mixed in.

In a small bowl, combine the flour, salt, baking powder, baking soda, and nutmeg. Add this to the wet ingredients, and mix on low until fully incorporated.

Divide the batter evenly into the 2 prepared loaf pans and bake for about 50 minutes, until a tester comes out clean. Take the bread out of the loaf pans and allow to cool completely before glazing (recipe below).

For the brown butter icing.

Brown the butter in a pan, just as described in step 2 for the bread (it may take a little less time because there's less butter) and allow to cool for about 10 minutes. Scrape the butter into a mixing bowl.

Sift the confectioner's sugar to remove lumps. Then whisk the vanilla into the butter. Next, whisk in confectioner's sugar until your reach a spreadable consistency.

Spread the icing onto the loaves, and allow to set for about 30 minutes before slicing.

Butternut Sage Scones

Ingredients You Need

2 cups (about 9 oz. or 255 grams) all-purpose unbleached flour (I use King Arthur)

6 tablespoons granulated sugar, plus more for sprinkling on top of scones

1 tablespoon baking powder

1/2 teaspoon kosher salt

1/2 teaspoon ground cinnamon

1/2 teaspoon fresh ground nutmeg

Scant ¼ teaspoon ground cloves

Scant ¼ teaspoon ground ginger

2 teaspoons finely chopped fresh sage (optional)

6 tablespoons cold unsalted butter, cut into small cubes

1/2 cup butternut squash puree (see below for directions)

1/3 cup heavy cream, plus more for brushing on top of scones

1 large egg

8 small sage leaves

Cinnamon drizzle, optional

How to Make

When measuring flour, fluff with a whisk, scoop it up with a spoon, sprinkle it into the measuring cup, and sweep off the top with the flat edge of a knife or spatula. But when I make scones, I always weigh flour, and bypass all that extra work.

FOR THE BUTTERNUT SQUASH: Pierce a medium butternut squash all over with a fork or tip of a knife. Place on microwave-safe dish and cook on high for about ½ hour, turning every ten minutes or so, until soft and mushy. Cut squash down the middle. If it's still hard in the middle, nuke it a little more. Scoop out seeds and pulp. Scoop out the soft squash, mash it a bit, and place in a mesh strainer over a bowl. Let drain for a couple hours, or overnight. Depending on the size of your butternut, you'll probably have extra squash, as this recipe only uses ½ cup. Make soup with the rest. Or double the scone recipe. And make a little less soup.

FOR THE CINNAMON DRIZZLE: mix 1 cup confectioner's sugar with ½ teaspoon cinnamon. Add 2 tablespoons warm water. Stir until smooth. I always do this by sight, so if too loose, add more sugar. If too thick, add more water. If not cinnamon-y enough, add more cinnamon. It should be thick like corn syrup. Set aside.

In the bowl of a food processor fitted with the chopping blade, place the dry **Ingredients You Need** and the chopped sage, and pulse to combine.

Add the butter, and pulse about 10 or so times. You want to retain some small pieces of butter. Don't blitz the heck out of it. Transfer the flour mixture to a large mixing bowl. If you've got some really large butter lumps, just squish them with the back of a fork.

In a large measuring cup, place the squash, egg and heavy cream. Mix well. Pour into flour mixture. With a dinner fork, fold the wet into the dry as you gradually turn the bowl. It's a folding motion you're shooting for, not a stirring motion. When dough begins to gather, use a plastic bowl scraper to gently knead the dough into a ball shape.

Transfer the dough ball to a floured board. Gently pat into a 6" circle. With a pastry scraper or large chef's knife, cut into 8 triangles. I use a pie marker to score the top of the dough circle and use the lines as a guide.

OPTIONAL BUT RECOMMENDED: Place the scones on a wax paper-lined sheet pan and freeze until solid. Once they are frozen, you can store them in a plastic freezer bag for several weeks.

Preheat oven to 425 degrees F. Place frozen scones on a parchment-lined sheet pan, about 1 inch apart. Brush with cream. Take the whole sage leaves, brush front and back with cream and place on tops of scones. Sprinkle tops of scones with sugar.

Bake for about 20 - 25 minutes, turning pan halfway through. They are done when a wooden skewer comes out clean. When cool, drizzle with cinnamon glaze.

Slather with clotted cream and fig jam, if you feel like gilding the lily. But if not, these are pretty darn good with just plain ol' butter, too. These are great the next day, warmed in the microwave for 15 - 20 seconds. They freeze really well, too, and can be reheated in a 350 degree F oven until warm. Enjoy!

BAKING TIPS: Last but not least, I highly recommend you get an oven thermometer, if you don't have one already. The success of quick breads like this depend upon a really cranking hot oven, and if your oven fluctuates, like mine does, then you can adjust your oven temp accordingly. Mine always runs cooler, so I crank it up until the thermometer reads the temp I want. Also, if you are baking less than a full batch, double up on your baking sheets, which helps prevent scorched bottoms.

Almond Cake with Oran

Ingredients You Need

2 eggs

1 cup natural yogurt

1 1/2 cups sugar (separated)

1/3 cup vegetable oil

1 cup all-purpose flour

1 cup almond meal

1 1/2 teaspoons baking powder

1/2 teaspoon baking soda

1/8 teaspoon salt

1 teaspoon vanilla extract

juice of 1 orange

2 teaspoons orange flower water

1/3 cup sliced almonds (not toasted)

How to Make

Preheat oven to 350 F. Butter and flour a 9 x 5 inch loaf pan. Combine eggs, yogurt, 1 cup sugar, oil, and vanilla.

Whisk together flour, almond meal, salt, baking powder, and baking soda. Add gradually to wet ingredients. Mix just until combined.

Pour the batter into the loaf pan, sprinkle sliced almonds evenly over the top, and bake for 40 minutes, or until a knife comes out of the center clean.

While the cake is baking, make the syrup: juice the orange and mix with remaining 1/2 cup sugar and orange flower water. Heat in small saucepan over stovetop until sugar has dissolved (5-7 minutes).

When cake comes out of the oven, let stand 10 minutes, then use toothpick to poke holes over the top and pour the syrup over. The syrup may puddle at the top- don't worry, it will sink in. Allow to cool before serving.

Mixed Berry and Walnut Crumble Bars

Ingredients You Need

1 cup walnuts, coarsely chopped

1/2 cup unsweetened coconut flakes (often labeled as coconut chips)

1 firm kiwi, peeled

2 cups to 2 1/2 fresh or frozen berries (do not thaw), any combination

1 teaspoon lemon juice

1 Zest of 1 lemon

1 1/4 sticks (10 tablespoons) unsalted butter, plus more for greasing the pan

1 1/2 cups all-purpose flour

1 1/4 cups old-fashioned rolled oats

1/3 cup granulated sugar

1/3 cup dark brown sugar, packed

1 teaspoon kosher salt

1/2 teaspoon baking soda

How to Make

Heat the oven to 350° F. Butter an 8-inch square baking pan and line the bottom with parchment paper.

Spread the walnuts and coconut flakes evenly in a small baking dish and toast for about 5 minutes, until just lightly browned. Let cool.

While the walnuts and coconut are toasting, coarsely grate the kiwi into a small bowl, making sure to catch the juice. Small remnants can be finely diced. Add the berries and lemon juice to the grated kiwi and stir to combine. Set aside.

Meanwhile, in a small skillet over medium heat melt the butter and cook until it turns brown and smells nutty, about 4 to 6 minutes. Be sure to stir frequently, scraping up any bits from the bottom so they don't burn. Take the pan off the heat and let cool slightly.

In a large bowl, whisk the flour, rolled oats, granulated sugar, brown sugar, toasted walnuts, coconut flakes, lemon zest, salt, and baking soda. Add the browned butter and stir with a wooden spoon until thoroughly combined.

Press 2/3 of the oat mixture in an even layer on the bottom of the prepared baking pan. Spread the berry-kiwi mixture evenly across the crust, then sprinkle with the remaining oat mixture.

Bake the bars for about 45 minutes, rotating the pan halfway through baking, until the top is golden brown and the berries are bubbling up around the edges. Transfer the pan to a wire rack and let the crumble bars cool completely. Cut into squares and serve. Bars can be kept in an airtight container on the counter for two or three days, if not longer. They'll soften as they age but retain their texture.

Apricot, Date, and Cashew Snack Balls

Ingredients You Need

1 cup cashews, walnuts, or almonds

Generous pinch sea salt

1 1/4 cups pitted Medjool dates (about 15 or 16 dates)

1/4 cup dried apricot

1 tablespoon almond butter

1/4 cup sesame seeds

1/2 teaspoon cinnamon

How to Make

Process the nuts and sea salt in a food processor fitted with the S blade till the nuts are coarsely ground.

Add the dates, apricots, almond butter, sesame seeds, and cinnamon. Keep processing the mixture until it's starting to stick together a bit. When you can squeeze a handful and it sticks together nicely, you're done.

Roll the mixture into balls that are about 1 inch in diameter. Store in an airtight container for up to two weeks in the fridge or a week outside the fridge.

Triple-Chocolate Olive Oil Brownies

Ingredients You Need

5 ounces dark semisweet or bittersweet chocolate (at least 65% cacao)

2 teaspoons (5 grams) instant espresso powder

1/4 cup (about 80 grams) chocolate syrup, preferably dark

1/2 cup (110 grams) extra-virgin olive oil

2 teaspoons (8 grams) vanilla extract

2 large eggs

1 cup (198 grams) granulated sugar, plus 1 heaping tablespoon for sprinkling (about 13 grams)

1 teaspoon (heaping) (8 grams) kosher salt

1/2 cup plus 3 tablespoons (82 grams) all purpose flour

1/4 cup plus 2 tablespoons (33 grams) Dutch-processed cocoa

1 large pinch flaky sea salt

How to Make

Heat oven to 350°F. Line an 8-inch square baking pan with parchment paper. (No need to grease— the brownies will take care of that for you while they bake.)

Melt the chocolate in a medium-sized heavy saucepan over a low flame, whisking constantly to prevent any from sticking to the bottom and burning. (You can do this over a double boiler if you prefer.) Remove from heat when there are just a few tiny lumps left, then whisk to finish melting. Add the espresso powder and syrup to the saucepan, and whisk.

To the same saucepan, add the olive oil and vanilla. Whisk. Add the eggs, and whisk until the mixture is smooth. Add the sugar, salt, flour, and cocoa powder, and whisk thoroughly enough to combine and ensure there are no lumps hiding in the batter, but then stop. (Over-mixing will lead to tough brownies—not what we're going for!)

Pour the batter into the prepared pan, sprinkle with the remaining heaping tablespoon of sugar all over, and top with a pinch of flaky salt. Bake until the brownies start to pull away from the sides of the pan and the middle looks puffed up and no longer liquid-y, about 30 minutes. (They won't look fully baked, but they'll set more as they rest.)

Allow the brownies to cool completely in the pan, then cut them into 1-inch squares. For the neatest-possible cut — since they're so gooey — you can pop them into the refrigerator for 15 minutes before slicing.

Yogurt & Berry Tart With a Pecan Crust

Ingredients You Need

1 1/2 cups raw pecans

1 tablespoon honey, more to taste

2 tablespoons unsalted butter, cold, cut into small chunks

1 cup (approximately) yogurt (preferably full-fat)
I think mascarpone cheese would also be yummy

2 pints or so fresh raspberries (you could also use
other berries, or sliced stone fruit)

How to Make

Heat your oven to 400° F. Put the pecans in a food
processor and pulse until you have a coarse,
crumbly meal, making sure to stop before you
blend it into a nut butter!

Transfer the pecans to a bowl and blend in the
honey I use my fingers then rub the chunks of
butter in with your fingers. Press this mixture into
a 9-inch round tart pan (it should fill the bottom
and come just a little way up the sides) and put the
pan on top of a rimmed baking sheet to catch any
oil that may leak out as it bakes.

Bake in the oven for about 12 minutes, until browned and toasty. Remove from the oven and allow to cool completely. Then, spread the yogurt into the crust and top with berries. You can serve immediately or keep the tart, covered, in the fridge for a few days, though the crust will become more fragile as it sits because it will absorb moisture from the yogurt. But it still tastes great!

Frosted Coffee Fingers

Ingredients You Need

1 cup light brown sugar, packed

1/2 cup unsalted butter

1 extra large egg

1/2 cup hot black coffee

1 1/2 cups sifted unbleached all-purpose flour

1/2 teaspoon baking soda

1/2 teaspoon Rumford's baking powder

1/2 teaspoon cinnamon (I use Vann's Saigon Cinnamon)

1/4 teaspoon fine sea salt

1 tablespoon instant espresso powder

How to Make

Preheat oven to 350° F. Butter a 13 x 17-inch jelly roll pan. Have all **Ingredients You Need** at room temperature.

Cream butter and sugar until fluffy. Beat in the egg.

In a separate bowl, combine dry ingredients. Add to the egg mixture alternately with the hot coffee. Mix well. Smooth the mixture in the prepared pan.

Bake in preheated oven for 13 minutes.

Allow to cool completely before frosting with the following icing: 1 tablespoon unsalted butter, melted 1 cup sifted confectioners sugar Enough orange juice to spread smoothly Mix butter and sugar. Add orange juice to make a thin but spreadable frosting. (The frosting will look almost translucent on the cookies.)

Cut into bars of the size you desire and watch them disappear!

Hazelnut & Caramel Cookies

Ingredients You Need

2 1/2 cups whole blanched hazelnuts

1 cup all-purpose flour

3/4 cup granulated sugar

1 stick cold, unsalted butter, cut into small pieces

1/3 cup heavy cream

1/4 teaspoon fleur de sel or flaky sea salt such as
Maldon

How to Make

Cut a sheet of parchment paper long and wide enough to cover the bottom and sides of an 8-inch square pan with 2 inches of overhang on all sides. Crumple up the parchment and straighten it out half a dozen times to soften it, so that it will fit into the corners without sharp edges. Line the pan with the parchment paper across the bottom and up the sides, pressing creases at the bottom and top edges.

In a bowl of a food processor fitted with a metal blade, process 1 cup of the hazelnuts, the flour, and 6 tablespoons of the sugar until the nuts are finely ground, about 2 minutes. Add the butter and process until the dough gathers around the blade, about 1 minute.

Scrape the dough into the prepared pan, press it with your hands into an even layer, and smooth the top with a small offset spatula.

Coarsely chop the remaining 1 and 1/2 cups of hazelnuts with a knife, aiming for mostly halves and leaving some whole.

In a medium saucepan over medium-high heat, bring the cream and the remaining 6 tablespoons of sugar to a boil, stirring frequently. Cook until it is thick enough to coat a spoon (running a finger down the back should leave a clear track), 3 to 5 minutes. Take the pan off the heat, immediately add the chopped nuts, and stir to coat them evenly. Use a spoon to distribute the nut mixture evenly over the dough, pressing lightly on the nuts with the back of the spoon to level them. Sprinkle the fleur de sel evenly over the surface. Freeze the dough, uncovered, until firm, 30 to 40 minutes.

Meanwhile, set a rack in the middle of the oven and preheat the oven to 350°F. Line a baking sheet with parchment paper.

Using the parchment overhang as handles, lift the dough out of the pan and transfer it to a cutting board. Using a large heavy knife, cut the dough into 5 equal strips in each direction to make 25 squares. Arrange as many cookies as you can fit on the prepared baking sheet, leaving about 1 1/2 inches all around them. Keep the rest of the unbaked cookies in the refrigerator.

Bake until the tops are caramelized and the hazelnuts are golden brown, 26 to 28 minutes Set the sheet on a wire rack to cool for 10 minutes, then transfer the cookies directly onto the rack to cool completely. Repeat with the remaining cookies.

The cookies will keep in an airtight container at room temperature for up to 5 days.

Vegan Dark Chocolate-Gingerbread Thumbprint Cookies

Ingredients You Need

Candied Ginger

1 cup coconut sugar, plus 3 tablespoons

2 cups water

1 3-inch piece of ginger, peeled and sliced into coins about 1/8-inch thick

Cookies & Chocolate Ganache

1 1/2 cups oat flour (store-bought works best) (180 grams)

1/2 cup (68 grams) super-fine almond flour

1/2 cup (72 grams) coconut sugar

1 teaspoon (4 grams) baking powder

2 teaspoons (6 grams) ground cinnamon

1 tablespoon (7 grams) ground ginger

1/4 teaspoon (1 gram) ground nutmeg

1/4 teaspoon (1 gram) ground cloves

3/4 teaspoon (3 grams) kosher salt

7 tablespoons (77 grams) refined coconut oil, melted

6 tablespoons (132 grams) blackstrap molasses

4.2 ounces Hu Simple Dark Chocolate (2 bars), roughly chopped into shards

3 tablespoons unsweetened coconut cream

How to Make

Make the candied ginger: Combine 1 cup coconut sugar with 2 cups water in a small saucepan, and heat over a medium low flame, stirring every minute or so, until the sugar dissolves (a few minutes total). Add the ginger coins and let it come to a rolling simmer for about 30 to 35 minutes, stirring every few minutes, until the liquid starts to bubble and cook down into a thick syrup. Drain the ginger pieces (you can reserve the syrup to use in cocktails later!), and toss them in 3 tablespoons of coconut sugar, then set aside in the refrigerator to cool and dry. This can be done several days in advance—just be sure to cover the candied ginger coins in the fridge. (You'll only need 14 of them for the cookies; save the extras for snacking.)

Heat the oven to 350°F. Line two baking sheets with parchment paper.

In a large bowl, combine the oat flour, almond flour, coconut sugar, baking powder, cinnamon, ginger, nutmeg, cloves, and salt. Whisk to thoroughly mix. Add the coconut oil and molasses and mix together with your hands or a wooden spoon until a moist ball of dough forms.

Divide the dough into 14 roughly equal pieces. Roll each into a ball. Arrange evenly on the prepared cookie sheets, and use your thumb to make a deep indentation in the center of each, almost down to the cookie sheet but not quite. (If the sides around the thumbprint start to split, just pinch them back together to create a retaining wall.) Chill the cookie sheets in the freezer for 15 minutes, then place into the oven. Bake for 14 minutes, peeking after 10 minutes to check on your indentations — if they're starting to fill in, briefly pull out the trays and press the indentations in with a teaspoon before returning to oven. Once you remove them from the oven, press down the centers one final time as they cool on their tray.

While the cookies are cooling, make the chocolate ganache. In a small saucepan, heat the coconut cream until melted and just barely simmering around the edges. Remove pan from heat and add the chocolate shards. Stir to combine until the chocolate has melted. Use a spoon to fill the centers of the cookies, and top each well of chocolate with one piece of candied ginger. Let sit at room temperature (or pop into the fridge for about 20 minutes, to expedite) until the chocolate centers have set.

To store, chill in a covered container for 2 to 3 days.

Cheese-Stuffed Figs Dipped in Chocolate

Ingredients You Need

20 ripe figs

1/4 cup (60 grams) soft creamy cheese such as ordinary cream cheese, fresh ricotta, mascarpone, or even a triple cream cheese such as Mt. Tam or Brillat-Savarin

5 ounces (140 grams) dark chocolate (any percentage—I usually choose a 62% or 70% chocolate for these), chopped

1/3 cup (45 grams) chopped toasted almonds or walnuts

How to Make

Rinse the figs and wipe them dry. Cut a short gash in one side of a fig near the bottom. Stuff with about 1/2 teaspoon of cheese. Smooth over the cheese so the fig remains shapely. Stuff the remaining figs and chill them for at least 30 minutes.

Put the chocolate in a small stainless bowl set in a wide skillet of almost simmering water; stir frequently until most of the chocolate is melted.

Remove the bowl from the water and stir until the chocolate is completely melted.

Line a baking sheet with wax paper. Make sure the figs are dry. Dip a fig into the chocolate and let the excess chocolate drip into the bowl.

Sprinkle the dipped fig with toasted nuts and set on the lined sheet. Dip the remaining figs. Refrigerate the figs until serving.

Vegan Chocolate Chip Cookies With Maple & Olive Oil

Ingredients You Need

2 cups plus 2 tablespoons (272 grams) all-purpose flour

1 teaspoon (6 grams) baking powder

1 1/2 teaspoons (6 grams) kosher salt

1/2 cup (102 grams) extra-virgin olive oil with a nice, mild flavor (avoid ones with a strong peppery flavor)

1/2 cup plus 2 tablespoons (180 grams) maple syrup

1 teaspoon blackstrap molasses

1 teaspoon vanilla extract

1/4 cup (24 grams) coconut sugar

1 3/4 cups (252 grams) dark chocolate chunks (note: use a vegan brand if you want to keep these fully vegan)

1 tablespoon flaky salt

How to Make

Heat the oven to 375F. Line two cookie sheets with parchment paper.

In a large bowl, whisk together all-purpose flour, baking powder, and kosher salt to combine and get rid of any flour lumps.

In a separate large bowl, whisk together olive oil, maple syrup, molasses, vanilla, and coconut sugar until fully combined and smooth—the mixture will look like slightly loose caramel. Add the dry ingredients and chocolate chunks, and use a wooden spoon or spatula to gently combine from the bottom and sides until there are no visible streaks of flour, but then stop. Over-mixing will make your cookies less tender. (Note: If you'd like to hydrate your flour as the original Ovenly recipe recommends, stick it in the fridge, covered, at this point for 12 to 24 hours. Or you can bake these right away.)

Grab a tablespoon or a scoop and divide the dough into heaping tablespoons, spaced out about 2-inches apart onto the baking sheets, with flat bottoms and domed tops; you should get between 24 and 26 portions. Sprinkle a little pinch of flaky salt over the top of each cookie.

Bake for about 13 minutes, until they've spread slightly (but they won't spread much) and there are slight striations starting to form around the edges — they won't look fully done, don't worry! Take them out of the oven and let cool a few minutes before attempting to move; they'll firm up as they rest.

Apple Chips

Ingredients You Need

2 medium, crisp apples (I like Jonagold), washed and dried

1/2 teaspoon ground cinnamon (optional)

How to Make

Heat the oven to 275°F. Use an apple corer to core the apples.

Set a mandoline to the 1/4-inch setting and slice each apple into about 15 thin slices. Or, slice the apples as thinly as you can by hand. Arrange the apple slices on two cooling racks set on top of baking sheets. (You can also used a Silpat-lined baking sheet.)

Sprinkle the cinnamon over the apple slices if using. Bake the apple slices almost dry, about 1 hour, flipping them over and rotating the baking sheets halfway through to ensure even baking. Cool the apple chips on a rack and serve or store in an airtight container for up to 2 days.

Multicolored Steamed Buns (Mantou)

Ingredients You Need

130 grams all-purpose flour

1 1/2 grams active dry yeast

50 grams granulated sugar

7 grams neutral oil, like grapeseed

80 grams milk, lukewarm

How to Make

Whisk together the flour, sugar, and yeast. Incorporate the milk and oil, stirring with chopsticks, a wooden spoon, or a spatula until you have a shaggy dough. If you're making two-toned swirl buns, you'll need to make two doughs, each with a different color.

Turn the dough out onto a floured surface and knead again until smooth, 4 to 5 minutes. You can also use a stand mixer fitted with the dough hook attachment. Place the dough in a large, greased bowl, cover, and let sit for 1 to 2 hours, or until doubled in size.

While the dough rises, cut out 12 squares of parchment paper, about 4- by 4-inches.

When the dough has risen, punch it down, transfer it it to a lightly floured surface, and divide it in half. Roll into long logs about 1 inch in diameter. Cut into 2- to 3-inch pieces, placing each one on a parchment paper square and on a baking sheet.

To shape swirl buns, roll each dough out into a rectangle, about 6 by 10 inches. Brush one dough rectangle with water (this will be the outer color), then place the other rectangle on top. Roll into a log, like you're making cinnamon rolls, then cut into 2- to 3-inch pieces. Turn them over if you'd like the swirl to be on top, or leave them standing up if you want the swirl to be side-facing. Proceed as usual.

Cover the baking sheet with a dish cloth or plastic wrap and let rise for 1 hour.

When you're ready to steam, bring a pot of water to a boil. Place the buns in the steamer basket with at least 3 inches of room between them (they're going to grow!). Steam for on low for 10 minutes, then lift the top and let the steam disperse for 2 minutes. Then recover the steamer and steam on high for 5 to 8 minutes, until the buns have grown in size and are shiny on top. (This method of steaming, while a bit more fussy, ensures smoother, glossier tops. If you're not in it for appearances, you can steam on medium for 13 to 15 minutes.)

These buns are best served piping hot. But never fear! You can freeze and reheat them easily. When the buns are fully cooled, seal them into a plastic freezer bag. To reheat, wrap with cling film or place in a sandwich bag and microwave for 45 seconds, or return to a steamer for about 2 minutes, until they've re-puffed.

TO MAKE PUMPKIN/ORANGE MANTOU, reduce the amount of flour to 110 grams (adding more as needed) and reduce the amount of milk to 30 to 35 grams. Whisk 70 grams of pumpkin purée into the milk and oil before incorporating it into the dry ingredients.

TO MAKE BEET/PINK MANTOU, reduce the amount of flour to 100 grams (adding more as needed) and reduce the amount of milk to 30 to 35 grams. Whisk 70 grams of beet purée into the milk and oil before incorporating it into the dry ingredients. (To make beet purée, we blended boiled beets with a little bit of milk—just 2 teaspoons or so—then passed the mixture through a fine mesh sieve).

TO MAKE MATCHA/GREEN MANTOU, reduce the flour to 125 grams. Whisk 6 grams of matcha in with the dry ingredients. Proceed as uaul.

TO MAKE CHOCOLATE/BROWN MANTOU, reduce the flour to 115 grams. Whisk 5 grams of Dutch-process cocoa powder in with the dry ingredients. Reduce the amount of milk to 70 to 75 grams.

www.ingramcontent.com/pod-product-compliance
Lightning Source LLC
Chambersburg PA
CBHW061037250726
48653CB00001B/139